Curing Yourself with Water

Knowing More about Hydrotherapy

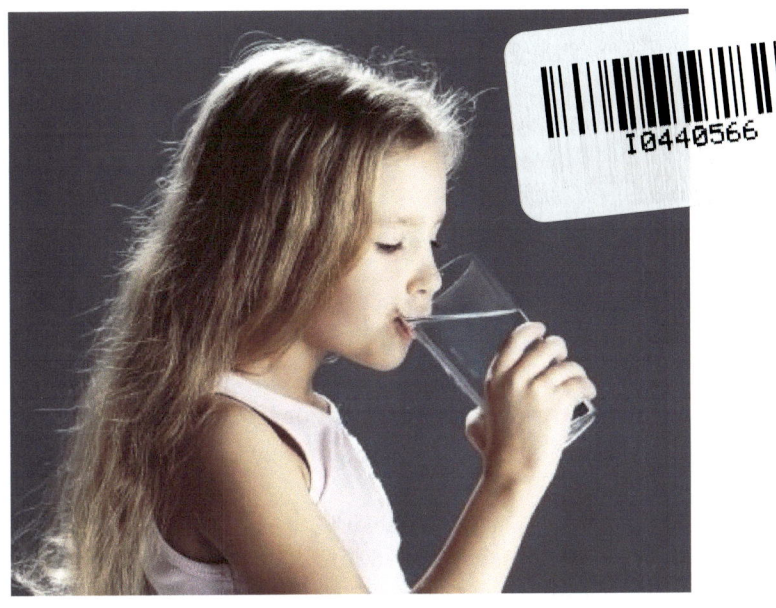

Dueep Jyot Singh

Healthy Living Series

Mendon Cottage Books

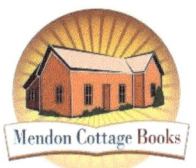

JD-Biz Publishing

Our books are available at

1. Amazon.com

2. Barnes and Noble

3. Itunes

4. Kobo

5. Smashwords

6. Google Play Books

Table of Contents

Introduction

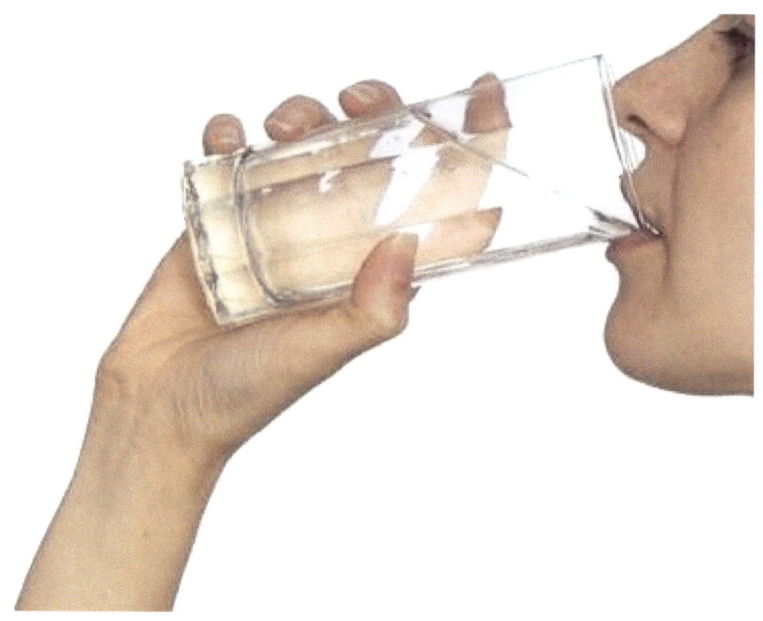

Two thirds of a human being's body is made up of water. Our body utilizes about 2600 g of water every day. The kidneys utilize 1500 g, the skin 650 g, the lungs 320 g, and 130 g of water is eliminated from the system every day. All this has to be restored through our food and the water we drink.

Naturally, that is the reason why the ancients always told us that the easiest way to keep healthy was to drink 2 ½ L of liquid every day. Not many of us do that because we think drinking water in such huge quantities would make us waterlogged!

So for all those people, who just cannot bear anywhere between 8 to 10 glasses of water every day, this book is going to tell them all about the beneficial uses of water. It is also going to tell them how they can take full advantage of the easiest element of nature available to them, and in such abundance to heal, to keep healthy, and to remain hydrated.

Do not do gulp down a glass full of water, the moment you grab it. Sip it down slowly – slowly, as if you have all the time in the world. This is so that if you are drinking cold or hot water, it takes a bit of while for the temperature to be regulated, to body temperature. By the time it reaches the stomach.

When I was young, I lived in a state, where the ladies of the house always boiled cumin seeds in the water, first thing in the morning, to make sure that there was absolutely no possibility of stomach afflictions and ailments troubling any member of the family which had to drink that water throughout the day.

In other parts of the country, people put basil leaves in water, and boiled that mixture to drink throughout the day, so that they did not suffer from any infections.

When Not to Drink Water

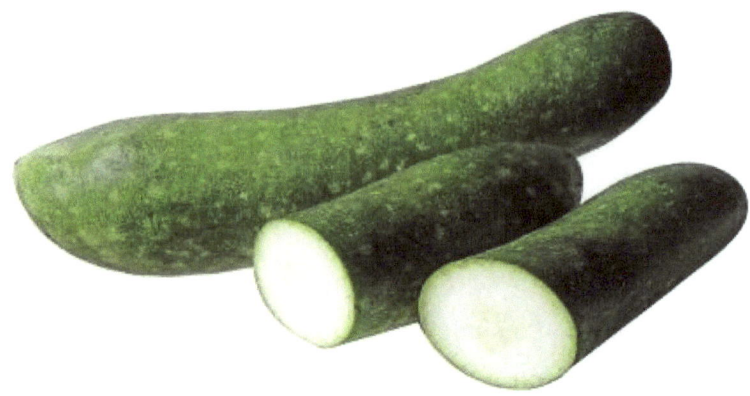

Cucumbers are already made up of 75% water. So you are not going to drink water, after eating them. Same goes for melons and cantaloupes.

I did not know that there were some rules and regulations about when you are not going to drink water. But according to the ancients, you do not drink water after eating hot food, cucumber, Armenian, melons, cantaloupes, the very first thing after you wake up, whether it is in the daytime, or at night, after cleaning your system while suffering from diarrhea, after drinking tea or milk, and coming in straight from a hot atmosphere outside.

I did not know this because the first thing I did, every morning for the past 10 years was to drink the water kept in a copper utensil, overnight next to my bed, and finish up 2 ½ glasses of it, the moment I opened my eyes.

This was excellent for clearing up my system within half-an-hour. However, I noticed that some of the ailments, supposedly clearing up my sinus and other chest related ailments which were supposedly going to be cured with that copper water still remained fixed permanently in their places of rest.

It is only after I got up, walked about a little, did a little bit of exercising and then drank that water, that I found out that the copper water had begun to do its magic work. I now do not have to worry about cold in the winter. Thanks to block sinuses, this was one of my chronic worries.

When Do You Drink Water

Now, this is when you are going to drink water. Do not drink it while you are eating your food because that is going to lower your digestive system's powers. Instead, if you really need to drink any water – just take a couple of sips, mid-meal. Drinking water immediately after you have finished the meal is going to make you put on weight.

Instead, drink a glass full of water, one are after you have taken a meal. This is going to increase the power of your intestines and your digestive system. People suffering from diarrhea should not drink water at all, when they are having their meals.

When Do You Drink Lots of Water

People suffering from high blood pressure, fever, sunstroke, urinary infections, constipation, and a burning sensation in the stomach should drink lots of water as often as possible.

How Do You Drink Water?

Let me tell you something interesting about this particular topic. As a child, I lived in some areas of the country where one never touched the rim of the glass to the mouth while drinking water! Supposedly, that glass would become impure and untouchable, and nobody else would drink from it, until it had been cleaned thoroughly.

Needless to say, the class system and the caste system has been prevalent in that area. For millenniums, people of one caste would never eat anything in utensils, which had been used by people of another caste. Historically, it is said about a king who invited another king to a banquet, at his palace. Both of them did not sit together to eat, both of them belonged to different warring castes.

The moment the other king and his retinue had gone out of the gates, the ruler host ordered all the utensils, which had been used in the cooking of the meals, including the utensils in which his guests had eaten to be thrown in the nearest pond. In fact, even today that pond is pointed out by tourist guides, who tell about great copper and silver utensils, buried under so much mud for hundreds of years!

Well, I was talking about drinking from a glass in the normal fashion. If any of my friends' mothers saw me drinking from a glass, like a normal human being, the glass was taken away, and wash thoroughly with salt and ashes before any member of their families were allowed to drink from that glass. Their justification was that infections could be passed on through unhygienic and infected saliva.

To me, I just considered all the actions of the adults around me to be thoroughly absurd and without any logic. I took it for granted that different peoples had different cultures and our job was to enjoy them and derive the most fun from some of their more out dated ideas.

That was the reason why, for millenniums, a person tilted his head back, and allowed to flow of water to pour into his mouth from a distance of about 12 inches away above his face. This was quite a perilous activity, because if that water flow missed its target, you were in for a cold face splash from your glass.

Nevertheless, children got used to drinking this way from childhood, and could also learn how to swallow that stream, without removing the source of flow from above their faces.

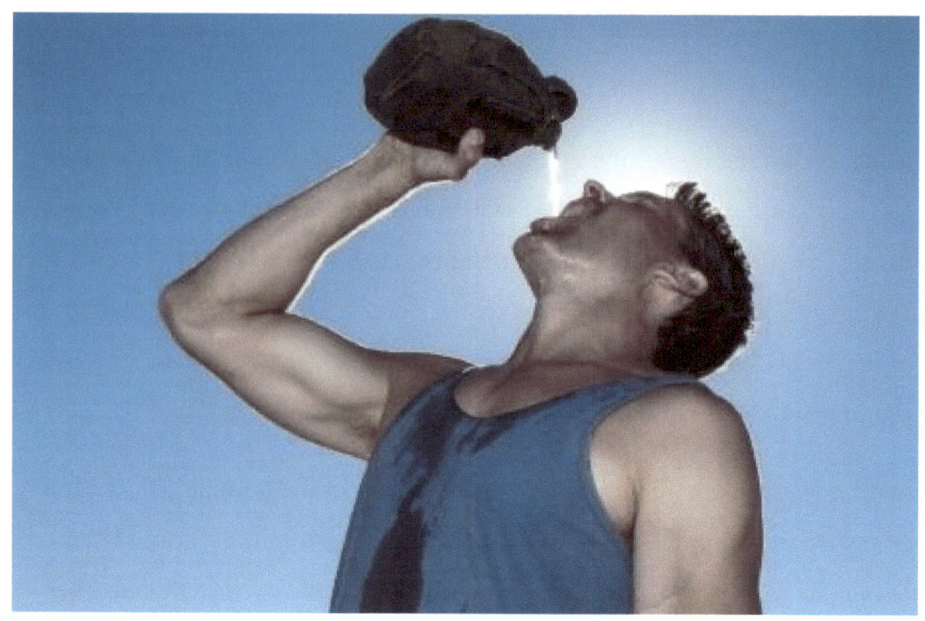

Even today, in many military training sessions, water is drunk from a canteen in this manner.

However, when I grew up, and came to another part of the country diametrically opposite in culture, and tradition from the area where I had spent my childhood, a naturopath told me, that this way of drinking water was definitely not healthy. Apart from water, you are also swallowing deep mouthfuls of air. This caused possible infections in the human digestive tract, as well as in the anal canal.

Also, the water with air, which has entered your system is going to cause constipation, acidity, and even nausea. So, according to him, the sensible way to drink water was to put your mouth to the rim of the glass, and sip it slowly.

How Much Water Do You Drink?

Some say eight to 10 glasses a day, and some say, do not drink so much and I still know others who talk about 8 L of water drunk every day, which I think totally appalling. Nevertheless, here is one formula which I am going to tell you, about how much water you need to drink, suited to your own individual body weight.

Take the weight of your body and multiply it by .55. This is the amount of water which you are going to drink throughout the day. For example, if you weigh 72 pounds that multiplied with .55 gives 39.6, which means 3 L 96 mL per day. If you do plenty of physical exercise outside, throughout the day, you will have to multiply it with 0.66.

Also, if you are feverish, and this infection is going to cause a lot of dehydration, drink plenty of water. This is your system, gets rid of the infections and toxins, and get your system moving again.

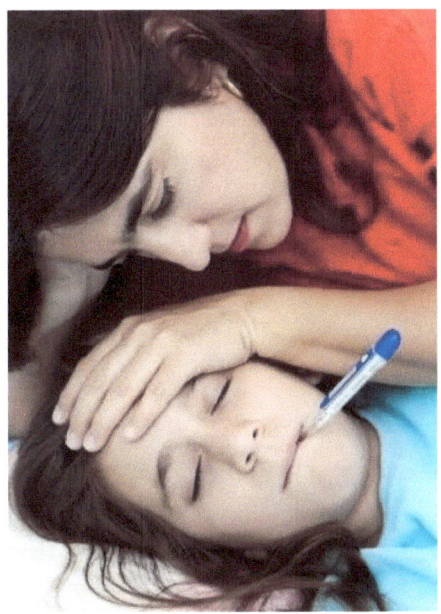

It is only a healthy body which control of the aftereffects of a fever and the vestiges of infection. Plenty of water is going to give you the strength to do exactly that.

How to Keep Healthy

According to the ancients, it was necessary that a human being drank water in little amounts, throughout the day instead of waiting for himself to get thirsty, before drinking huge glasses of water.

According to them three sips of water, often, drunk throughout the day kept the heart, body, mind, and soul; gentle and peaceful.

That is why the ancients woke up in the morning, said their prayers, and then drank three sips of water. The same was done when they said their prayers at night before going to sleep – three sips of water. According to them, this kept them healthy spiritually, physically, and mentally. For them, water in itself was an healing agent and cure for a number of ailments and prevented them from occurring.

Drink water, three hours before any meal or before any exercise, especially if you are going out for a walk. If you intend to indulge in any physical exercise, drink water, 2 ½ hours before doing that physical labor. That means that your body has enough of strength given to it by a well hydrated system, and provides this energy to your tissues and muscles.

Water is the 2nd element, which is going to help your body heal itself naturally. Naturopaths swear by water therapy. Water therapy is known as hydrotherapy in their circles. Not only is it an excellent stimulant, but it is also capable of reducing fever, a good antioxidant, and tones up your system considerably.

But before I tell you more about water therapy, I would like to give you some more ancient tips with which you can gain full benefits from water. Of course you are not going to drink water which is muddy, has impurities in it, or is from an open source outside like a river, or a pond. Any stagnant water should definitely be avoided, especially if you are on a hike and come across an open water source.

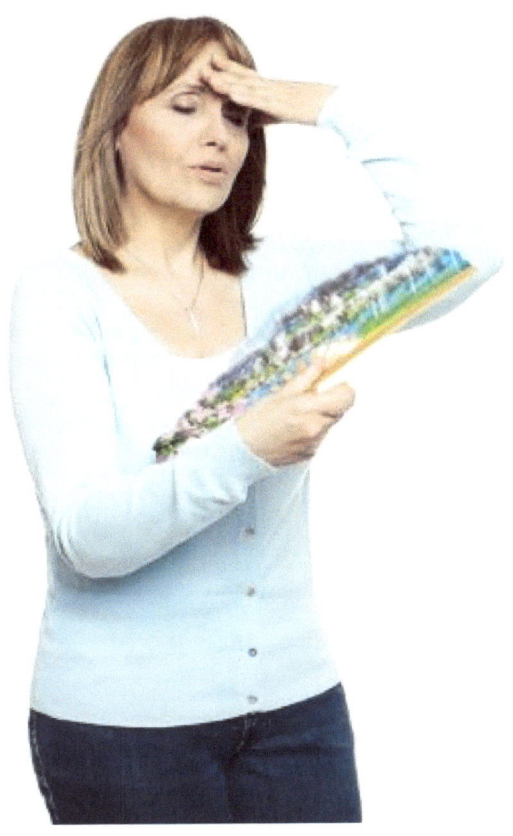

But hey, you are dying of thirst, and you need to drink some water. If you see life forms in it, and the water is flowing, you can take a chance of drinking it. But if it is still and stagnant, you are better off trying to look for another water source.

If the water is not pure, boil it, and filter it. That is going to get rid of a major part of the impurities. Do not drink too hot or too cold water. We have this nice habit of going straight to the refrigerator and chugging straight from the bottle. Not only is this terrible for our teeth, but doing this, when you are overheated, coming straight in the house from a terribly hot, sweltering summer outside, and there you are, you have opened yourself up to a bad summer cold and associated problems.

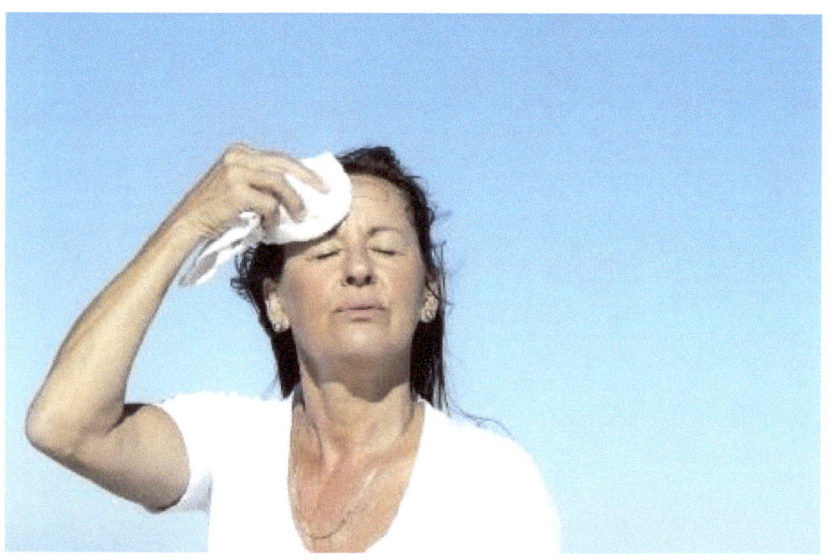

Dehydration and loss of water, especially in the summer are one of the main causes of heatstroke and summer ailments.

Believe it or not, many of the brands of the expensive mineral water which you buy in bottles off the supermarket shelves are often not as pure as they are advertised. In fact, once I managed to get into one of these factories where this water was being "manufactured!" It was then bottled as pure mineral water and sent all over the world under a very famous Brand Name.[1]

Here are the ways in which you can keep yourself healthy, just by drinking water. Drink four large glasses full of water, first thing in the morning, after you have got up and then some exercise, on an empty stomach. The ancients normally recommended anywhere between half a liter to 1 L of water on an empty stomach, but that is a bit too much for me and for you, in the initial stages.

Drinking less than 5 to 6 glasses a day is going to lead to constipation.

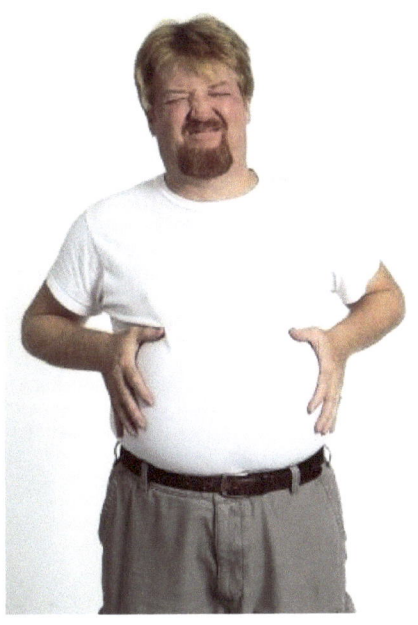

---

[1] Name Withheld. It is a multibillion-dollar industry. And I do not want them to screech libel.

You can increase the intake of water early in the morning, as time goes by. This is normally done without you brushing your teeth, washing your face, or doing your early morning ablutions.

This water is going to be placed at your bedside at night. Traditionally, it was placed in a copper utensil, so that it could absorb all the qualities of that metal throughout the night.

After you have drunk the water, you can go ahead with washing your face, brushing your teeth, showering, shaving, and so on. But do not eat or drink anything for one hour after you have drunk this water.

This water is cleansing your body of the toxins accumulated during the nighttime. It is also going to stop you from suffering from constipation.

Do not drink any water when you are eating your meals. If you have to drink anything liquid, you may take a couple of mouthfuls before or during your meal, or half an hour before a meal. But the ancients did not drink anything for 2 hours until after a meal, so that the saliva and the gastric juices could do their best work. The water that you drink during the meal is going to interfere with the gastric juices produced in your body during the digestion process.

You can also control your weight by drinking the juice of one lemon, and one tablespoonful of honey, in lukewarm water first thing in the morning. This is also excellent for your skin, keeping it well moisturized.

Keeping Your Eyes Healthy

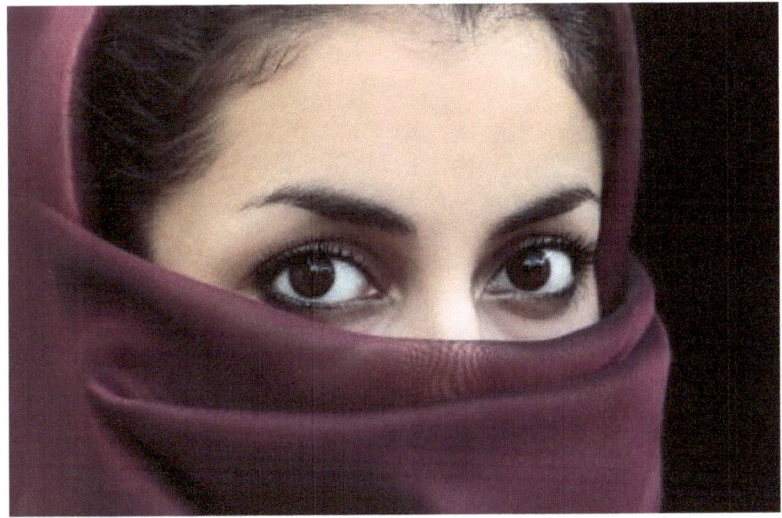

According to the ancients, after you took your food, you washed your hands with pure, clean water. Then you rub your hands/palms, and apply those wet hands on your eyes. If you did this every day, your eyes would never suffer from any sort of ailment and if there was some ailment ready to occur in your eyes, it would disappear.

According to me there is a very clear scientific explanation to it. You wash your eyes, and then you rub your eyes with the wet palms, cleaning them in the process too. Doing this, after every meal means less chances of infection through hands transmitted to eyes, and the ancients had a good way of getting people to wash their hands after a meal!

Hot Water Fomentation

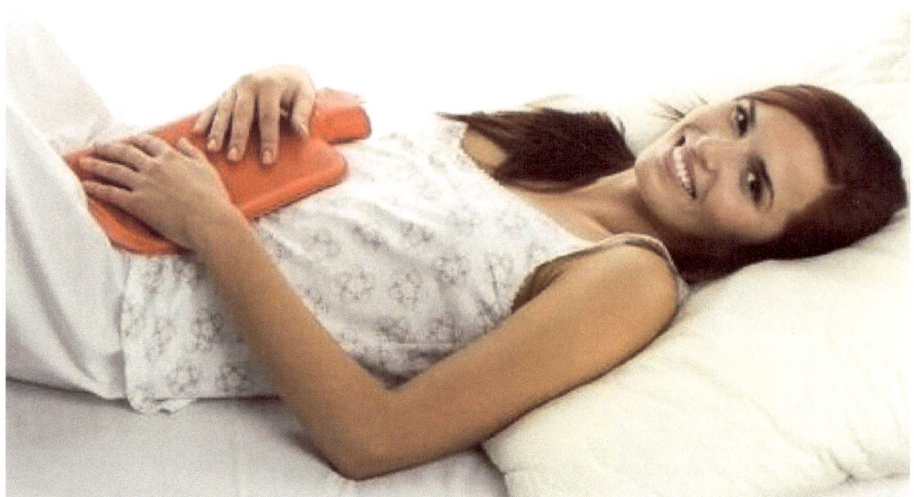

This is the best way in which you can get localized pain relief. Cover the affected region with a hot-water bag or a cloth dipped in hot water. This method of applying heat is going to result in the improvement of circulation and the reduction of pain. That is because the muscles have gotten relaxed.

Remember to wipe the parts subjected to this treatment, with a cloth dipped in cold water, after you have done the fomenting.

Pain relief can take anywhere between 15 minutes to 45 minutes depending on its intensity. You may also need to refill the hot-water bottle with water during the process. Make sure the water is not boiling hot.

Cold water fomentations are also excellent to keep the body cool, especially during summer.

I normally make a cold water foment by filling up my hot-water bottle three fourths with water and put it in the freezer. Four hours later, I have a frozen cold water bottle. Lovely to apply on heated skin, in the summer, especially after a hard day's work outside. Wrap it up in a piece of cloth, so you do not have to bother about the condensation.

This fomentation is excellent, especially when you have sprained any organ. You are going to do this on the second day after you have a sprain. You are going to put that affected part in hot water, and allow the heat to seep through and cure the injured tissues.

Healthy Bath

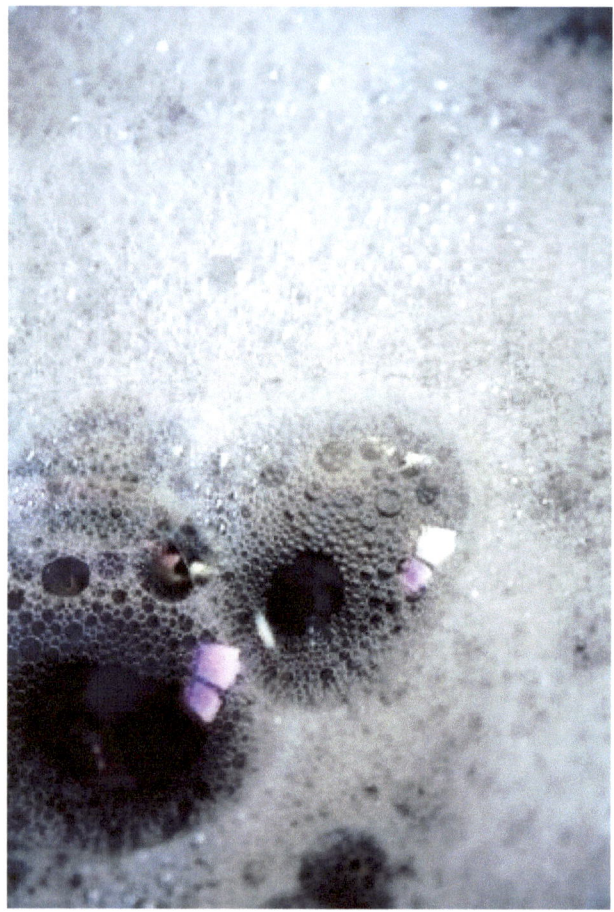

Apart from old people, and people were suffering and recuperating from fever, the ancients suggested having a cold bath instead of a hot water bath. My grandmother, being brought up in this stoic tradition used to wake up at Dawn every day, like her ancestors had done for millenniums and then bath in cold water, even though it may be 0° outside. Her son, my father, followed in her footsteps, and I used to shiver when I saw him coming out of the bathroom after a cold shower, of a cold December morning when I was watching the hot water geyser warming up for my daily shower.

Funnily enough, she never caught a cold, even though we thought cold and pneumonia would have been the aftermaths of taking cold water baths when it is snowing outside. But then, I believe, a very strong immune system, and a body accustomed since childhood to a cold water bath allowed her to be so stoic.

This was, of course, torture to grandma's grandkids who were really coddled and cossetted from day one. Nevertheless, the hot water baths had a detrimental effect on the skin, because it left it dry. So after we got out of our baths, we had to rub coconut oil all over our bodies and faces to moisturize the dry skin. Apart from that, we had to stand in the steaming bathroom for a while, for the skin to get accustomed to the change in temperature, before we walked into our bedrooms where the temperature was about 15° higher.

This abrupt change from hot to cold was conducive to future colds and chest infections.

So since childhood, we were told, close your eyes, jump into the bath, and you are not going to feel cold after the first 30 seconds! In fact, people who felt upset or feverish were immediately put in the cold bath because that shock in itself would get rid of all those symptoms.

Grandma never used soap while bathing, but used natural cleansing remedies like Clay, milk cream, oatmeal, and wheat bran as cleansing agents. These are the cleansing remedies which are still being used in many parts of the East, where expensive beauty creams, powders, lotions, and "lip reddeners" are still considered to be taboo to "good girls of good family!"

Do not entertain the mistaken notion that the use of expensive perfume soaps and very expensive beauty products are going to make you as beautiful as the superstars who endorse them. They have their own genetic make-up and so do you. Both are miles apart. So thinking that cleansing your skin with expensive beauty products is going to keep you young looking, and healthy, well, that is all a multibillion-dollar industry's propaganda working overtime.

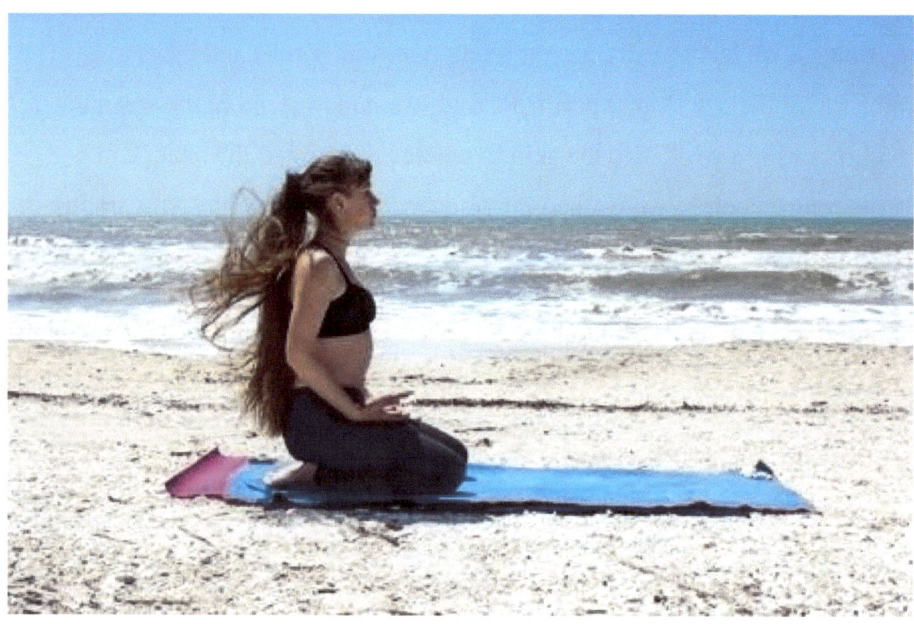

Too much exposure to the sun, without any proper adequate covering, and water, means a bad sunburn and possible sunstroke.

I remember suffering from a sunstroke while on official tour to the city where my parents lived. My temperature was more than 103°F, so the moment I walked inside the door, I staggered straight into the bathroom half delirious, and got under the shower with clothes and shoes still on with the whole family thinking I had gone bonkers.

I think I stood under the shower for the next 20 minutes, and then remembered to shut the door and change into my night suit. After that I slept for four hours in a semiconscious stupor. By the time I woke up, my sunstroke had gone, my fever had gone, and I was stoutly denying the fact that I would do something so stupid as to stand under a cold shower in my official uniform, without even taking off my shoes.

So the moment you begin to feel feverish, get under a cold shower, and stand there for 20 minutes.

About two decades ago, my father, being an avid mountain climber decided to go on a trek on a pilgrimage 4500 feet above sea level. He was in his 60s at that time, and walking 14 miles up a steep slope, his leg muscles got cramped. Luckily, there were mules, which took him to his destination where the priests immediately told him to go and have a bath in the holy water pool next to the place of worship.

Now, that pool was ice cold, full of glacier water. But it becomes a matter of pride, especially when you are on a pilgrimage, you dunk yourself in icy cold water at a temperature of 5° below, just to show everybody that you are full of religious fervor. Every single pilgrim was doing exactly that!

I am astonished that none of them died of shock. Nevertheless, when my father came out all rosy and glowing out of the cold water dunk, the muscular cramps had gone!

When he recounted this to me, when he came back – incidentally taking to his bed with a terrible cold – I told him that the scientific explanation was that the body was so shocked at the change of temperature that it told the circulation to act quickly and bring the body temperature back to normal and heat it up again. That fast blood flow got rid of all the cramps in the muscles.

So this is the reason why the ancients did not bother much about muscular pain and cramps. They just took a dive into the nearest cold water, fresh icy source, notwithstanding.

Hip Baths

These are extremely effective to cure ailments in the liver, stomach, intestines, kidneys, spleen, and other digestive organs. If you are suffering from abdominal pain or cramps, take a hot water hip bath. Place a napkin which has been dipped in cold water on your head and scalp during this time.

You can alternate between a hot water and cold water hip bath after spending 2 minutes in each tub to gain even more benefits of this natural curing process.

A hip bath has a very special type of tub. It is about 30 inches long and 20 inches wide. It is also known as a sitz bath, because the patient sitz in it, no pun intended, immersed to his hips.

This URL can give you some more information about hip baths.

http://www.wisegeekhealth.com/what-is-a-hip-bath.htm

So alright, I did not bother to buy a hip bath. I just went to the nearest caterers and asked them whether they could sell me a round metal/plastic tub in which they collected used plates, cutlery, and crockery after the feasting was done.

They had plenty of them, exactly right for what I wanted. I could "accordion" myself into that tub with my knees outside, and the upper portion of my torso nice and dry.

So once you have your bathtub installed, fill it up with lukewarm water to a depth of 8 – 10 inches [up to 25 cm.] Now drink a glass of warm water and sit in the tub, with your abdomen and parts of your thighs submerged in the water. The upper trunk portion and the legs are going to be outside your tub.

Keep massaging the abdominal region with a little bit of pressure, using a coarse and thick towel. A hot water hip bath in the winter should take about 15 minutes. In the summer, you can enjoy a cold water hip bath for about half an hour.

Make sure that you dry yourself completely after a hip bath. You are going to take it on an empty stomach. Do not eat anything for about one hour after you have taken this bath. Let nature do her own curing.

Steam Baths

The Romans swore by steam baths. Half of the work of the state was done in these ancient steam baths, when all the Senators and the patricians used to gather every morning, and get their slaves to massage them with olive oil or beat them with twigs to get there circulation moving again.

In ancient Rome, steam baths were made through pipelines of boiling hot water hitting ice cold water of the bath and everybody boiling himself in the ensuing steam. Nowadays, specially designed cabinets or steam boxes are used in steam baths. They are rather expensive, so spas which use them regularly prefer investing in such boxes. And that is what you enjoy during your sauna bath in that spa.

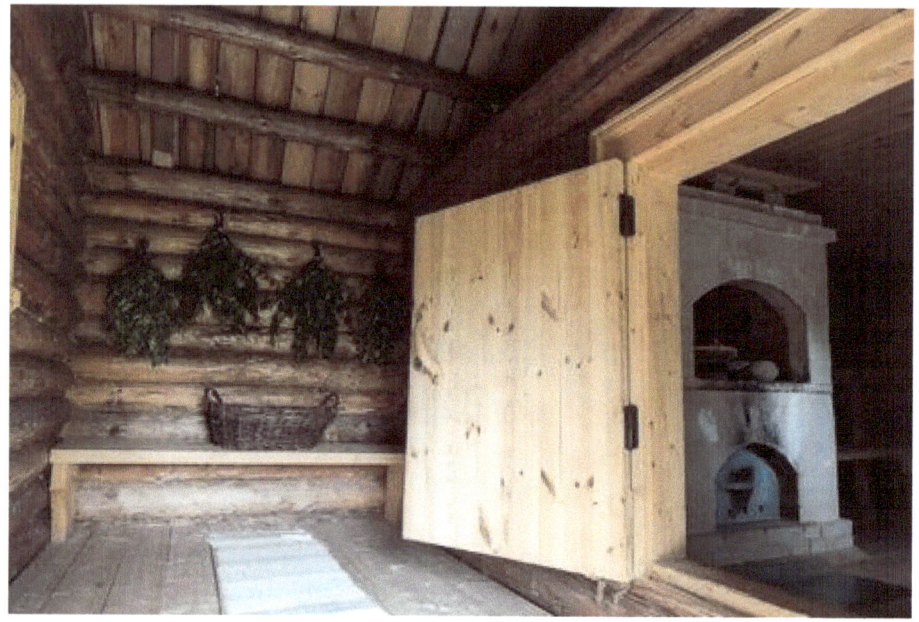

Traditional sauna baths have birch brooms or brooms of other herbs to apply on your body during the scrubbing process.

The steam bath should normally be done once a week. This gets rid of all the toxins accumulated in your body, opens up the pores, and also helps clean the surface of your body properly, getting rid of the dust and grime.

Getting rid of the toxins is normally done by drinking lots of water and to prevent the accumulation of toxins in the body, you need to eat seasonal fruit with your food, green leafy vegetables, and food items with lots of fibers in them.

Toxin poisoning is normally going to take its form of symptoms like nausea, no appetite, lethargy, headache, and an upset system.

Many of us take the symptoms for granted, thinking them to be the symptoms for some other ailment. What we do not know is that our body is slowly and steadily getting poisoned with the toxin accumulation. This is the reason why. Apart from steaming to get rid of the toxins, we need to drink lots of water, and boost up our leafy vegetable and fruit intake in our diet right now.

Steam Baths for Weight Loss

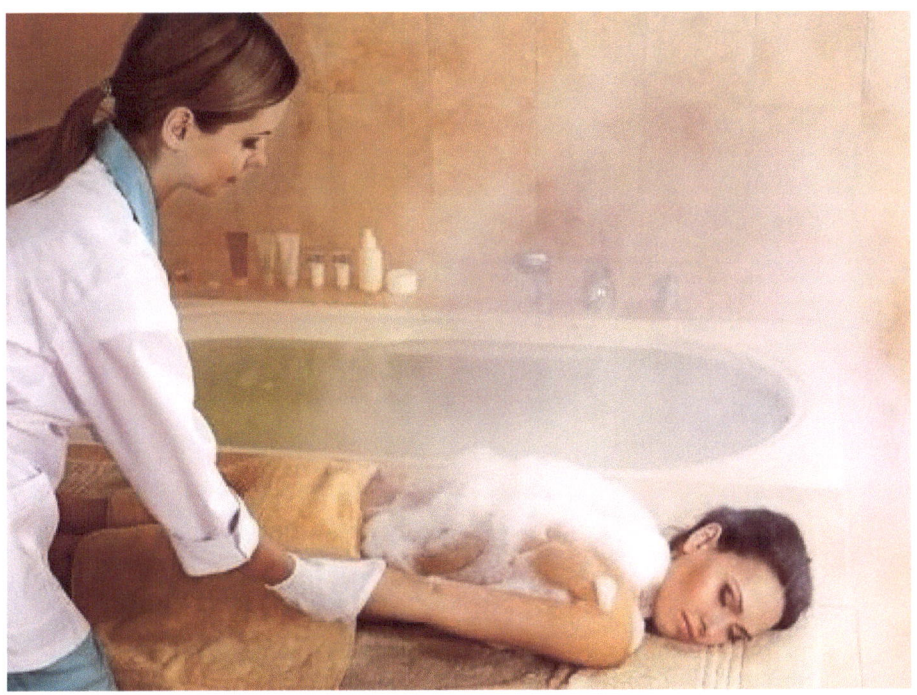

Spas have their own steam baths, also known as hammams or Turkish baths.

In ancient times, it was supposed that subjecting your body to hot steam and then plunging into a cold bath would be enough to get rid of excess weight. Sometimes, that is justified, because it is possible that our body has retained some water because it is in a dehydrated condition.

So it is going to get rid of all that water, when it gets plenty of water into its system.

Here is one tip you may want to try if you think that you are retaining water. Stop drinking all those eight glasses of water, I advised you at the beginning of the book. This is going to get some of the excess water out of your system. But make sure that you do not find yourself totally dehydrated. Use some common sense here. The moment you feel that you need to drink water, go drink it.

Start drinking lukewarm water instead. If you take a glass full of lukewarm water, before you have any sort of meal, that is going to prevent you from stuffing yourself on the table. Take 125 g of water, and boil it. Allow it to cool. When it is lukewarm, put 3 tablespoons full of lemon juice in it, and 2 tablespoons full of honey. Drink this early in the morning on an empty stomach to make sure that you are not dehydrated, and to give you energy.

Try this out for two months, and you are going to see a different visible positive change in your weight problem.

However, when you are doing this treatment, you think you may be able to get away by eating fatty foods, well, the answer is no. You will have to eat a light meal. Eat this light meal, once a day. Try eating bread from which the brand has not been removed, whole wheat. Start eating more green vegetables, both in raw form and in cooked form. In the evening, just eat fruit because you are not going to starve yourself, are you.

Do not drink any water with the meal. Remember, you drank a glassful of lukewarm water, before the meal, in order not to feel so hungry. Drink the lukewarm water, again, one hour after you have had your meal. Try to stop drinking tea, coffee, fatty foods, and sweet items.

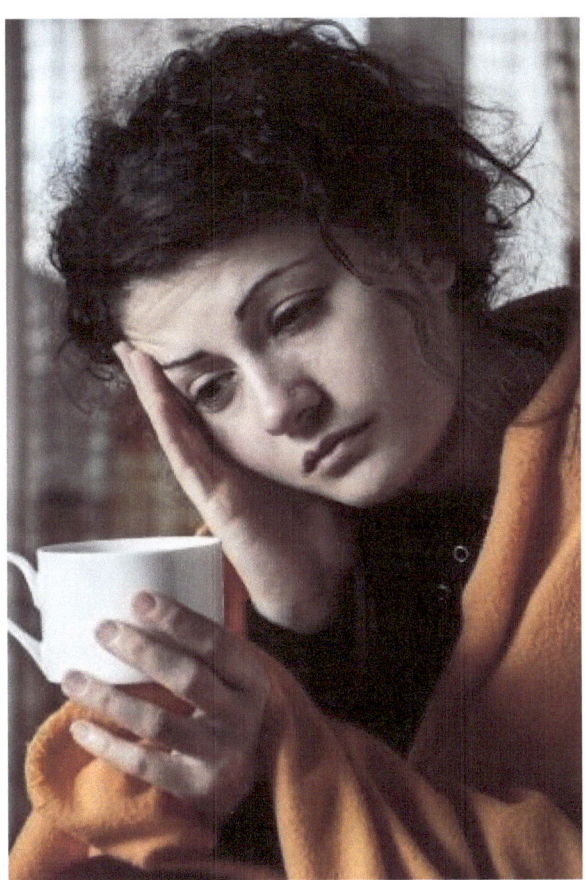

With both your meals, fruit and light lunch – you are going to drink one cup of really hot water, about as much hot as you can bear to sip. Let me tell you one amusing thing here. I seriously have rarely drank tea or coffee in my life, because the idea of a person burning his mouth three times a day and then asking for his caffeine fix, every four hours seems rather silly to me.

There must be some sort of masochism in a person who drinks boiling hot tea and coffee and enjoys it. So, if you are a boiling hot tea or coffee drinker, drink water at the same temperature. Funnily enough, you are not going to like drinking this hot water. You think it really hot! I still cannot make out that particular psychological quirk.

You are going to drink this hot water in little sips, as if you were drinking tea or coffee. You can always take a mouthful of cold water in the middle of your meal. In this manner, the ancients managed to get rid of all that excess fat, with the drinking of hardware. But remember that they had a very active life outdoors, full of exercise and also, they drank and ate moderately. They also ate lots of fruit and vegetables.

Do not do this hot water for more than two months ever. This is the time it is going to take for that fat to melt down.

A well-known naturopath of the 19th century named Doctor Lucas recommended that his fat patients take three glasses of hot water and add a little bit of salt to them. This water was then boiled and allow to cool down. One glass was drank early in the morning, on an empty stomach, the other in the afternoon, and the third, before you went to sleep.

He was a very fashionable medical practitioner in the 19th century, and his patients swore by his remedies. Along with that, he asked them to go riding in the fresh air, early in the morning and get some exercise. Their food would be regulated and limited only to fresh vegetables and fruit.

See how this sensible man managed to get his patients to go out and exercise and eat sensibly. No wonder they found a distinct weight loss within two months.

Breakfast for Weight Loss

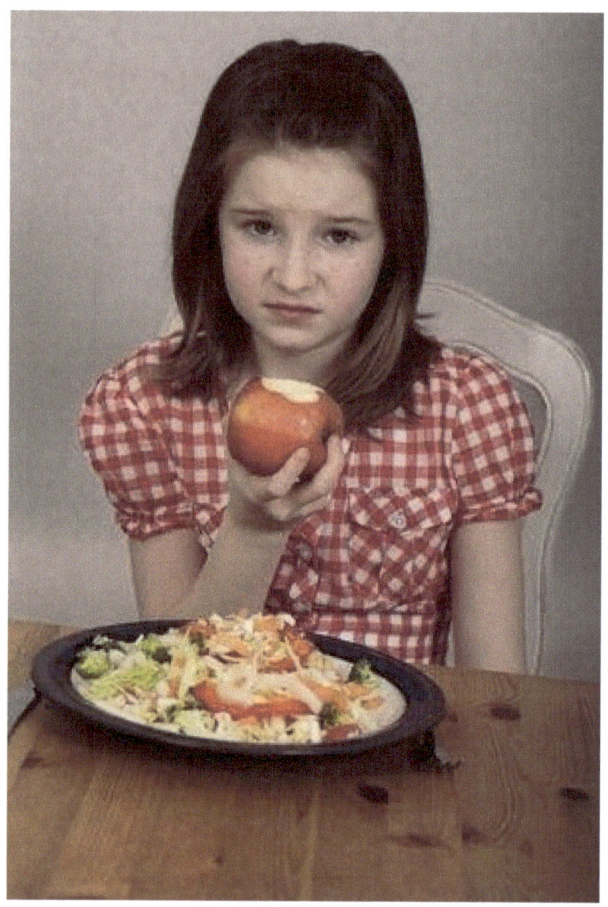

Eat apples, which have not been peeled, and carrots. You can also grate them together and eat them. This grated combination should be eaten early in the morning, for breakfast on an empty stomach, with a happy mood. Eat as much of these as you can do so. Or at least 200 g if you can manage them. Do not eat anything else, after eating this grated mixture for at least two hours to allow them to digest and assimilate in your body.

This is an excellent weight loss remedy.

On the other hand, if you are losing weight, and you want to put on weight, you are going to eat this same mixture, after having your lunch. Strange, how different timings can have different effects on your body.

Steam Boxes

These baths in the form of steam boxes began to be more well-known and popular in the Victorian era, when spas started introducing them in mountain resorts for tourists. However, they were universally known to eliminate toxins from the body for thousands of years. In fact, this was a known method in which the ancient Romans brought down their weight with an increase of the metabolic rate of their bodies.

This bath is taken when the stomach is empty. Drink a glass of warm water and enter the cabinet with minimal clothing. Apply a towel dipped in cold water around your head to keep it cool. After all, matters are going to steam up in a while.

This is normally done under the supervision of an attendant, who keeps sprinkling cold water on your head to keep it cool.

Steam from either a steam pipe or from any other steam source is let into the cabinet. If you find yourself getting lightheaded or dizzy, come out of the steam bath immediately.

When sufficient perspiration has been formed, – 10 to 15 minutes, – get out of the steam bath and take a cold bath immediately. Your body is going to feel young and rejuvenated.

Do not take this steam bath, if you are a heart patient, are expecting, or have high blood pressure.

If you are a DIY sort of person, this URL may prove interesting, especially when it is so easy to make.

http://www.instructables.com/id/Steam-bath/

Hot Water Cures

Hot water is excellent for getting rid of weight, indigestion, constipation, colitis, diarrhea, cold, just infections and throat infections, fever, respiratory infections, etc.

If you have eaten lots of spicy and rich fatty food, drink one glass of hot water. This is going to prevent any adverse effects of that food not being digested properly. Drinking hot water regularly is going to cure you of all your ailments, given above.

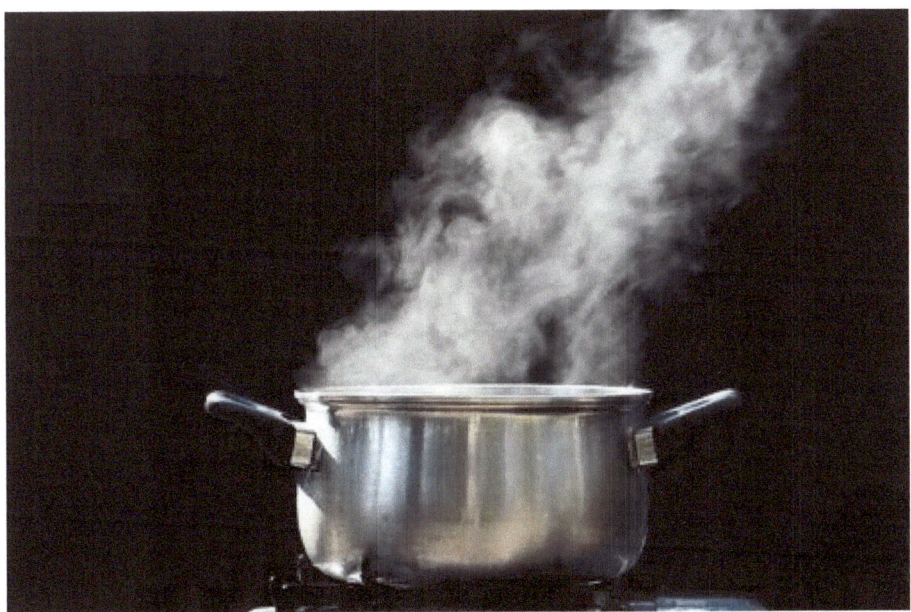

Take a glassful of hot water, and imagine that you are boiling it as you would boil your daily cup of tea. Sip this, to get rid of cold, cough, sinus problems, laryngitis, sneezing, headaches, constipation, and indigestion. If you put the juice of half a lemon in this hot water after you have put it in your glass, so much the better. This is going to increase your appetite and enhance your digestive properties.

If you want to make sure that you do not suffer from cold or cough this winter, make it a habit to drink hot water, early in the morning.

When we were children, my grandmother massaged us with warm oil in the summer and allowed us to bake. In the winter, she massaged us with a towel dipped in hot water, and after that we were put in the winter sun to gain full benefits of the rays.

People who are suffering from gout and pain in the joints or swelling in the joints can benefit a lot, by drinking lots of hot water. This is going to get rid of all the toxins, by clearing up the urinary system. That means the uric acid build up in the system is going to listen and thus you are not going to suffer from gout. That is such a logical solution, that I wonder why not many people follow it.

Also, if you are suffering from pain in the waist, drink lots of hot water. However, if you are drinking it cold because you do not like to drink this hot water, put five leaves of basil in it or two small cardamoms ground up and then boil the water. This water is going to be drank throughout the day. This means that if you boil it in the morning, you are going to finish it by the evening. And if you boil it in the evening, you have to drink it throughout the night, till the next morning.

In this way, you can also drink lots of cold water with basil and cardamoms in it. This is going to help cure pain in the waist.

If you are suffering from pain in the full body, or swelling of your feet, put the affected area in lukewarm water in which you have added a little bit of salt, allow that portion to soak for half an hour and you are going to find a distinct reduction of swelling and pain.

Apart from this, if you keep drinking hot water, you are not going to suffer from constipation, or flatulence. Also, you will not suffer from swelling of the stomach – ascites – and cramps. Your liver is also going to get stronger.

Let me tell you about another side effect benefit of drinking lots of hot water, which I just found out by chance. Drinking hot water means that you are not going to have black circles under your eyes anymore. Also, your skin is going to glow because all the toxins have been cleared out of your system.

Hydrotherapy

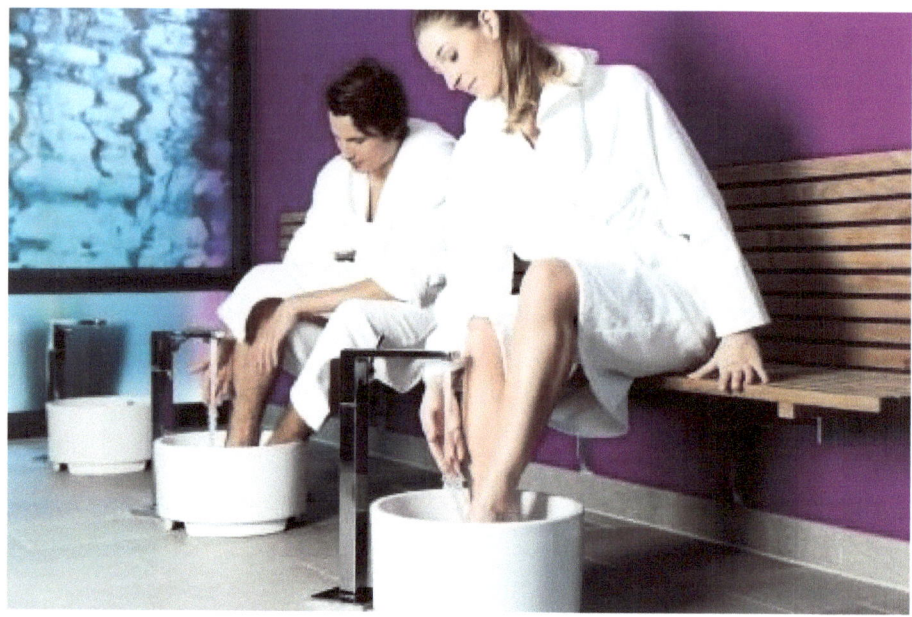

Different hydrotherapy processes include steam baths, hot foot baths, enemas, hip baths, fomentation, and irrigation of the stomach. Many of these procedures are still being used in spas, while others are considered to be old-fashioned and obsolete – including enemas, hip, and foot baths.

Naturopathy advocates regular bathing. Gone are the days when the idea of "bathing harms the skin" was spread in many parts of the world, especially in medieval times. At that time, body odor was masked with sweet smelling perfumes.[2]

Naturopathy includes keeping your body clean through regular bathing. Not only does this wash away all the dirt, but the scrubbing process stimulates circulation and relieves fatigue.

People who perspire freely should bathe twice a day. Lukewarm water or cold water is best for bathing purposes. Hot water bath may be very pleasant, but they take away the precious moisture from your skin. On the other hand, a cold water bath is very stimulating because it boosts up the circulation.

Place a napkin or a thick cloth dipped in cold water and wrung on your stomach. Now bandage it with a dry bandage. Allow it to rest for one hour. This is an excellent traditional cure for acidity, problems of the liver, ulcers, and even cramps.

.

---

[2] It is said that Princess Caroline of Brunswick – in keeping with the times – had such a displeasing body odor that her other fastidious husband, the future George IV, [notorious as Prinny and having learned to keep clean in body and clothing from his friend Beau Brummell] had said, "we may have married that woman, for the sake of England, but being near her is a punishment. "

She also did not like him much. So she encouraged that attitude by not changing her outer or inner garments for 6 months at a time. They did manage to have one child, Princess Charlotte, but it is well known that his wedding night was the only time when George came near his "legally wedded wife" for the sake of the throne of England.

Hot Foot Baths

This is extremely easy to set up, to reduce congestion of water in your upper torso. You are going to use fairly hot water in a bucket. Fill the bucket up, about three quarters, and pick up a woolen blanket.

Now place the bucket in front of a chair, sit down and wrap the blanket around you. Have a napkin dipped in cold water ready at hand to place on your head.

Immerse both feet at the same time. You are going to start perspiring within the next 15 to 20 minutes. When you have totally sweated it out, literally and figuratively and find yourself drenched with sweat stop your bath immediately. Make sure that you keep your head cool by sprinkling cold water on the napkin on top of your head.

Ladies should make sure that their hair is dry and unconditioned, when taking this bath. Wet, half dry, and just shampooed hair is going to help you to catch a cold, really quickly.

After you have finished bathing, wipe your body with a cold, wet cloth. Then lie down for 10 minutes.

So your legs are all red. That is because the circulation in that particular area has increased. Your feet are going to reach their normal state of color and tan in about half an hour. Unless, of course you are Superman and plunged your feet into boiling hot water and allowed them to cook. That is when you need the help of a doctor.

If you have not managed to bring up a sweat in the next 15 to 20 minutes, that means the temperature is less. Take out your feet, and add 4 glasses of boiling water into the bucket. Then dip your feet in and wrap the blanket again around you.

Your blood pressure is going to decrease during this procedure. That is why you need to lie down because you are going to feel all dizzy and weak.

That is why I repeat, people with high blood pressure, heart problems, and expectant mothers, should not take this therapy.

Conclusion

This book has given you plenty of well researched and time-tested remedies, with which you can cure yourself of common ailments with the help of just ordinary water.

So reach for your glass of cold water right now or hot water, if you are trying to get rid of all the ailments and toxins beleaguering your body.

Live Long and Prosper!

Author Bio

Dueep Jyot Singh is a Management and IT Professional who managed to gather Postgraduate qualifications in Management and English and Degrees in Science, French and Education while pursuing different enjoyable career options like being an hospital administrator, IT,SEO and HRD Database Manager/ trainer, movie , radio and TV scriptwriter, theatre artiste and public speaker, lecturer in French, Marketing and Advertising, ex-Editor of Hearts On Fire (now known as Solstice) Books Missouri USA, advice columnist and cartoonist, publisher and Aviation School trainer, ex-moderator on Medico.in, banker, student councilor ,travelogue writer … among other things!

One fine morning, she decided that she had enough of killing herself by Degrees and went back to her first love -- writing. It's more enjoyable! She already has 48 published academic and 14 fiction- in- different- genre books under her belt.

When she is not designing websites or making Graphic design illustrations for clients , she is browsing through old bookshops hunting for treasures, of which she has an enviable collection – including R.L. Stevenson, O.Henry, Dornford Yates, Maurice Walsh, De Maupassant, Victor Hugo, Sapper, C.N. Williamson, "Bartimeus" and the crown of her collection- Dickens "The Old Curiosity Shop," and "Martin Chuzzlewit" and so on… Just call her "Renaissance Woman" - collecting herbal remedies, acting like Universal Helping Hand/Agony Aunt, or escaping to her dear mountains for a bit of exploring, collecting herbs and plants, and trekking.

Check out some of the other JD-Biz Publishing books

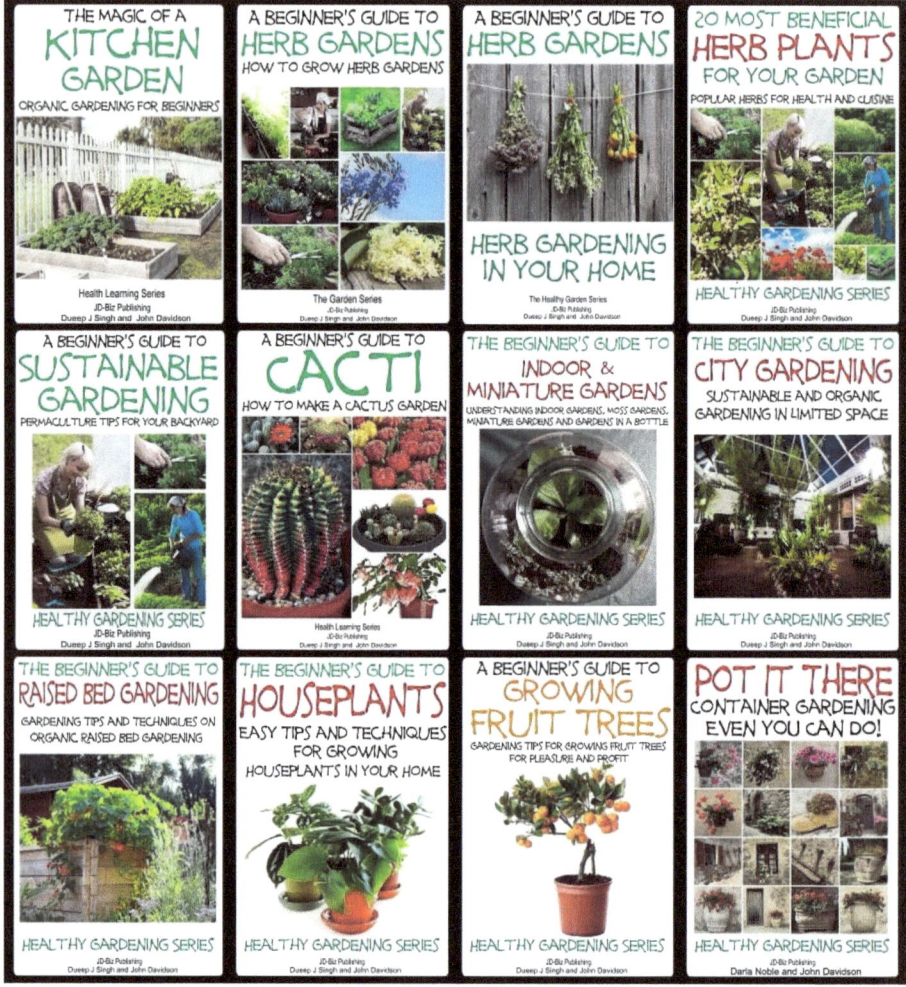

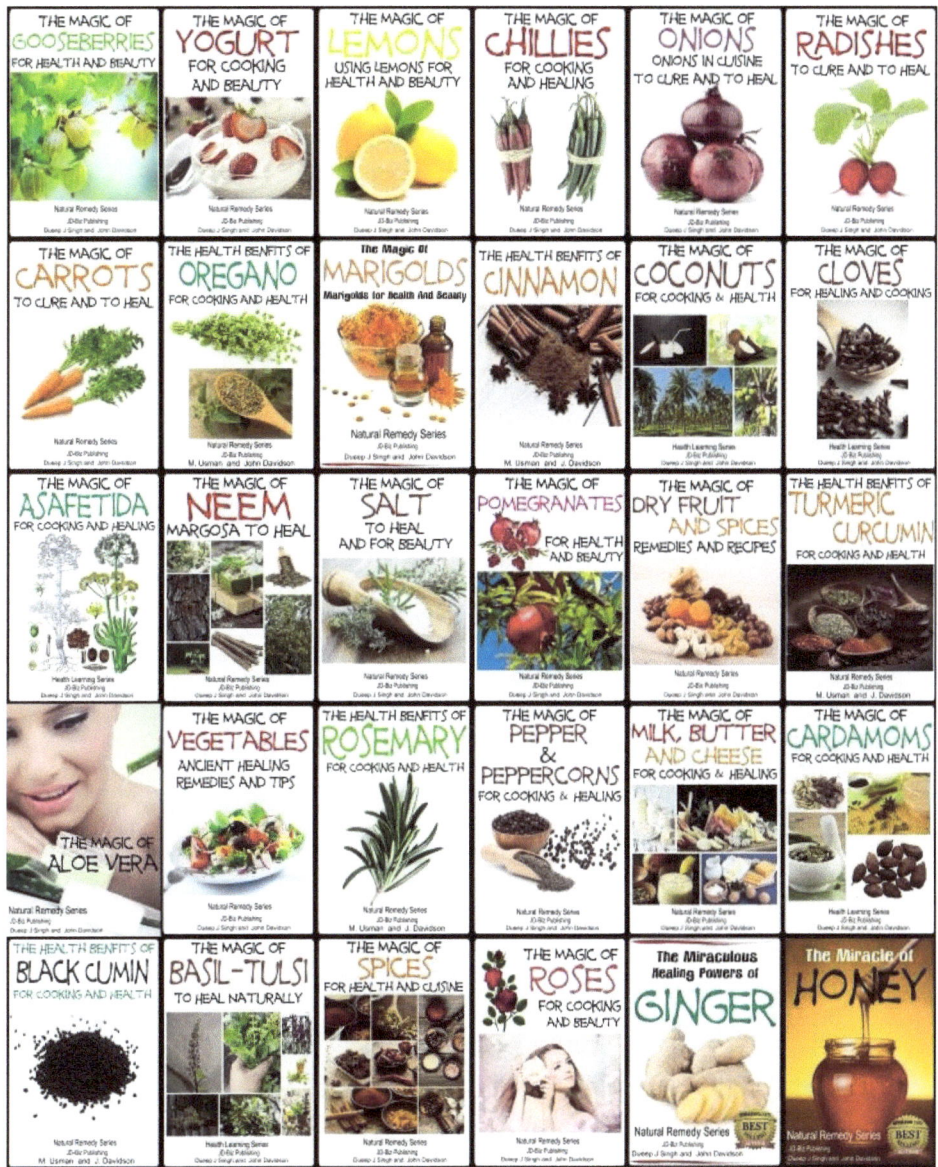

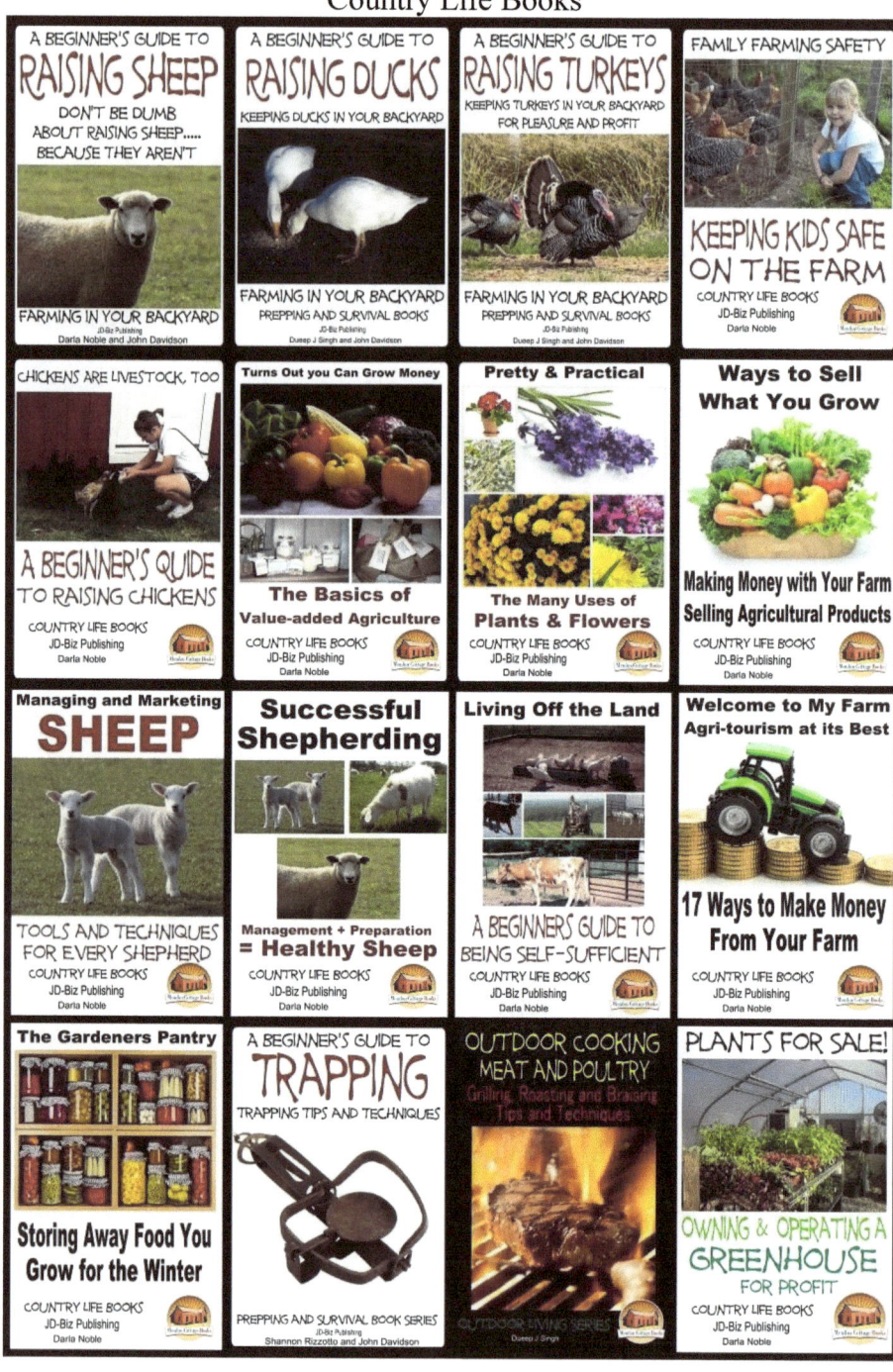

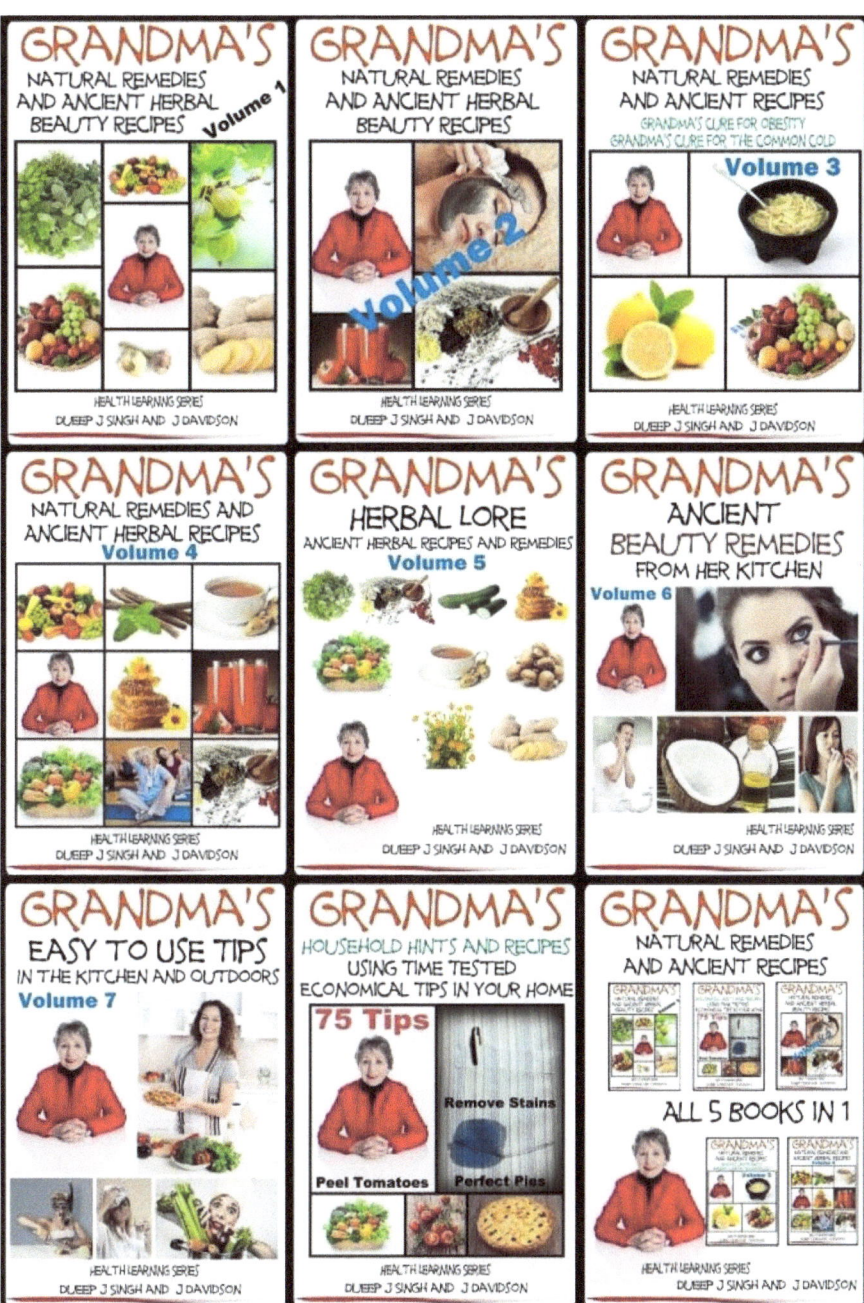

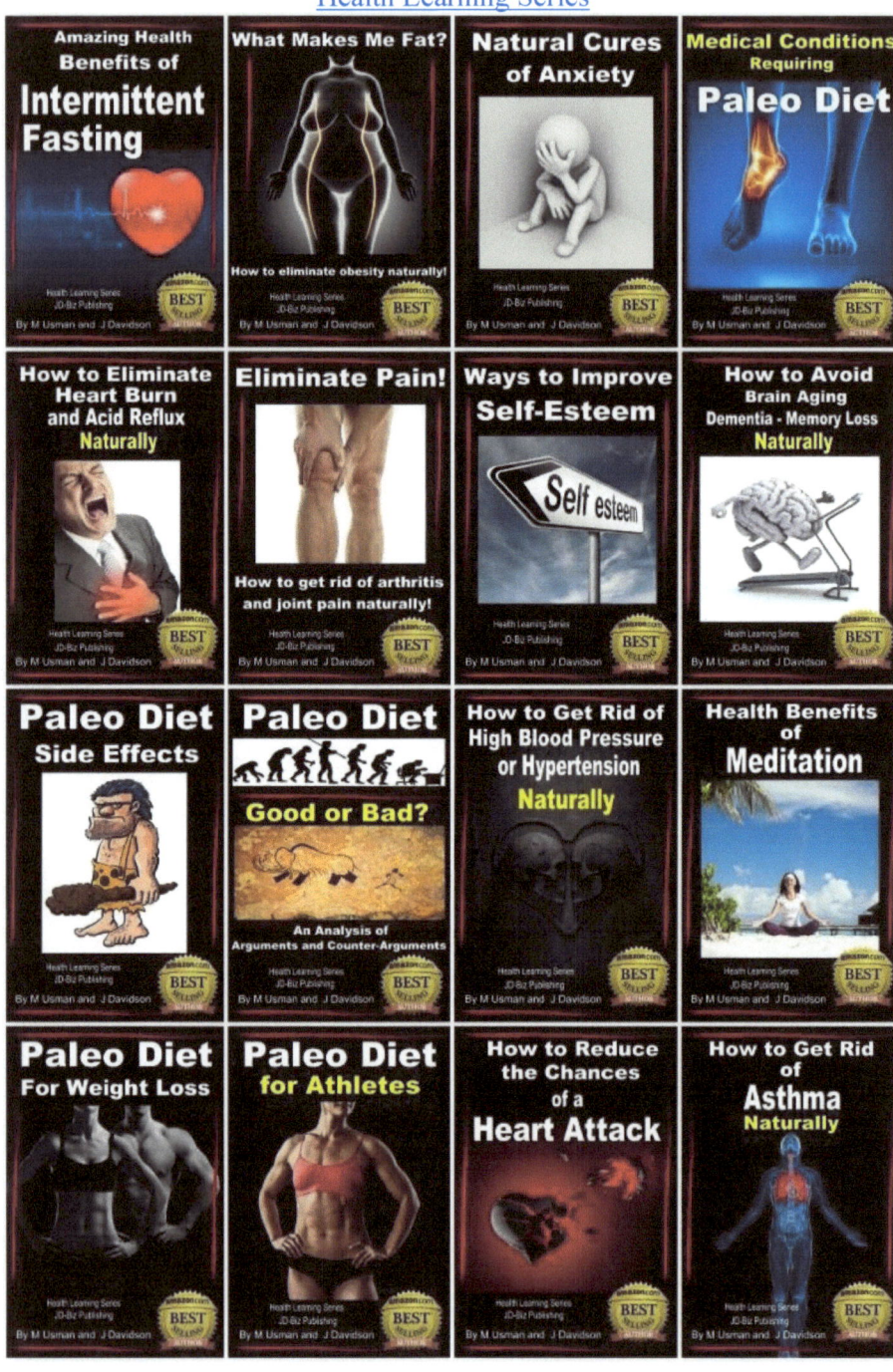

Amazing Animal Book Series

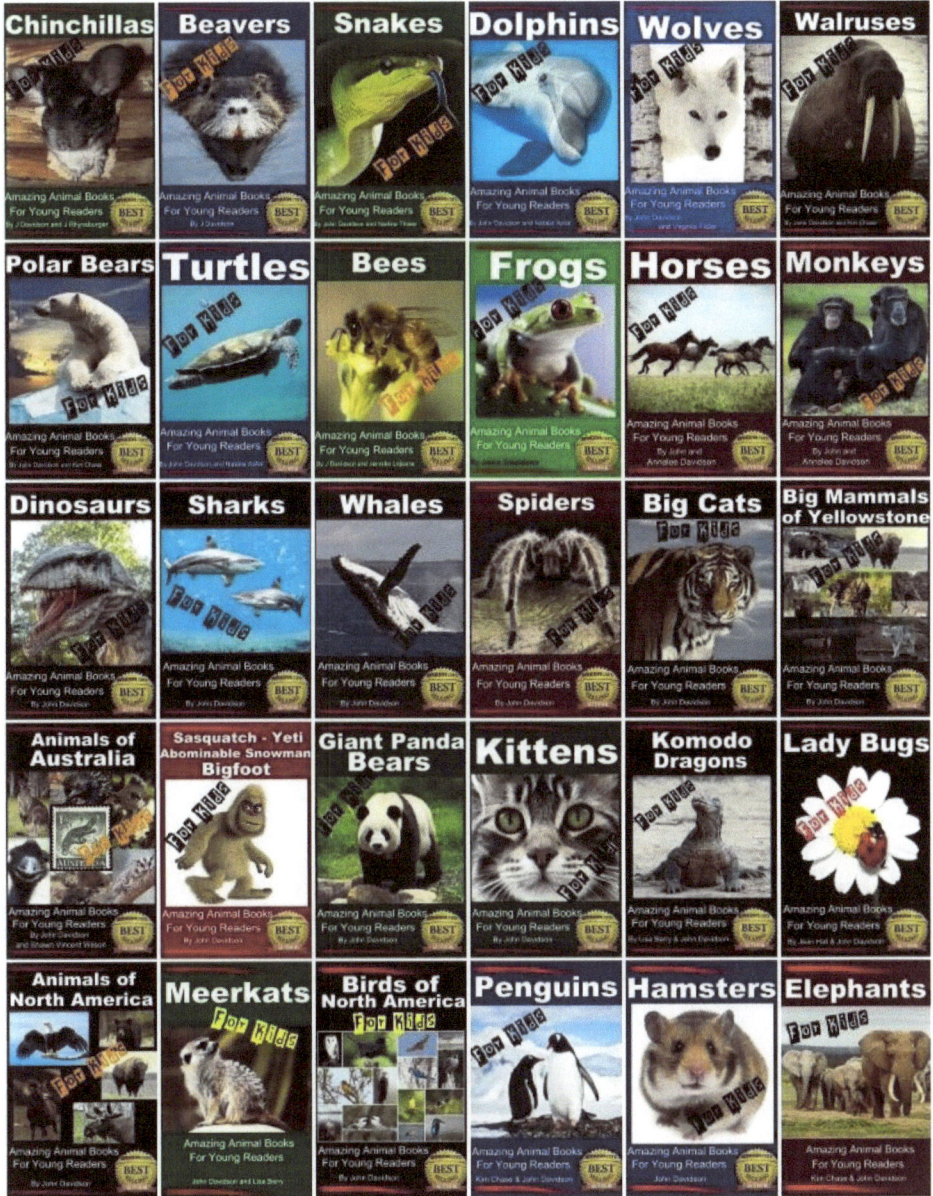

Learn To Draw Series

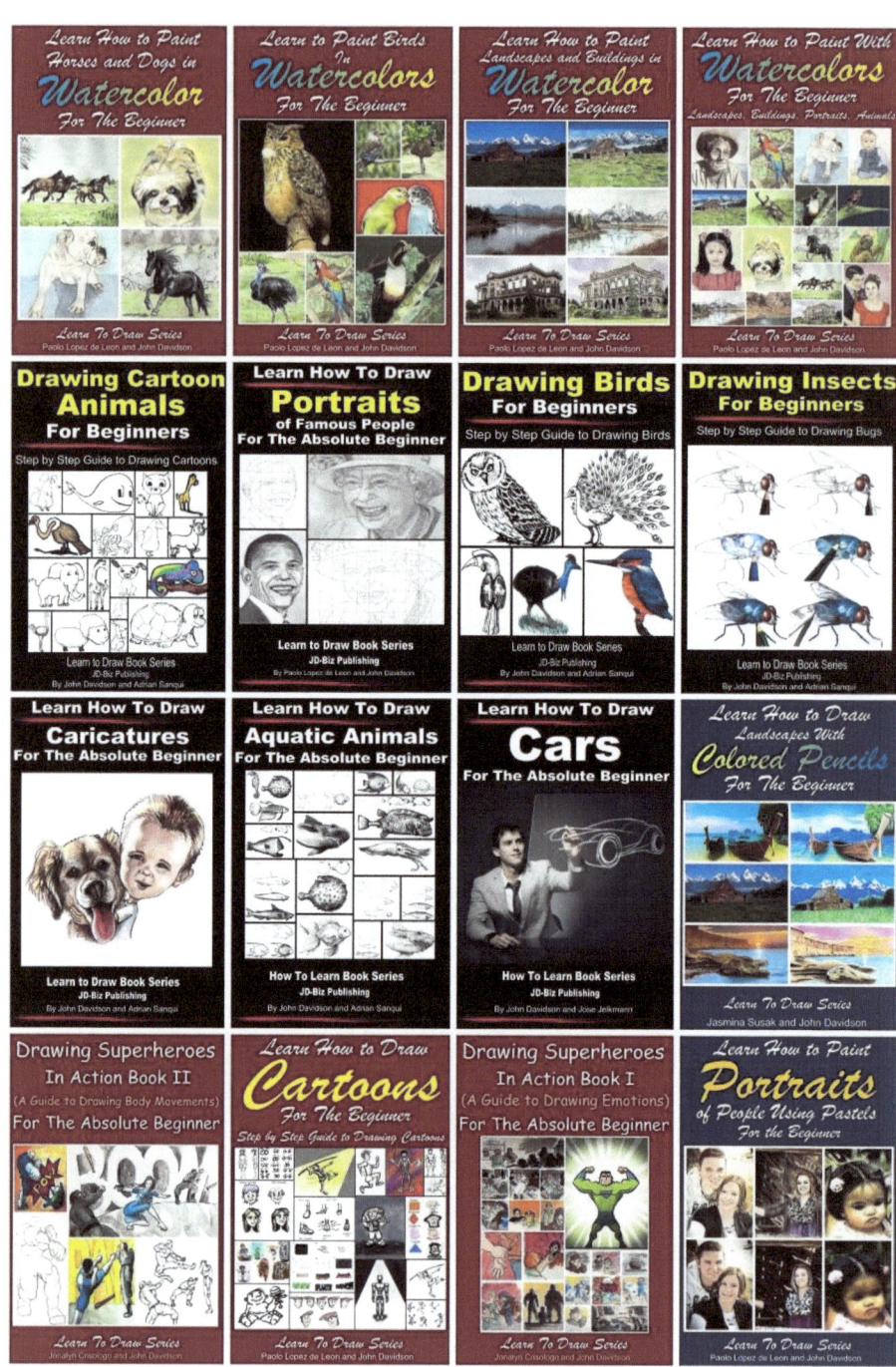

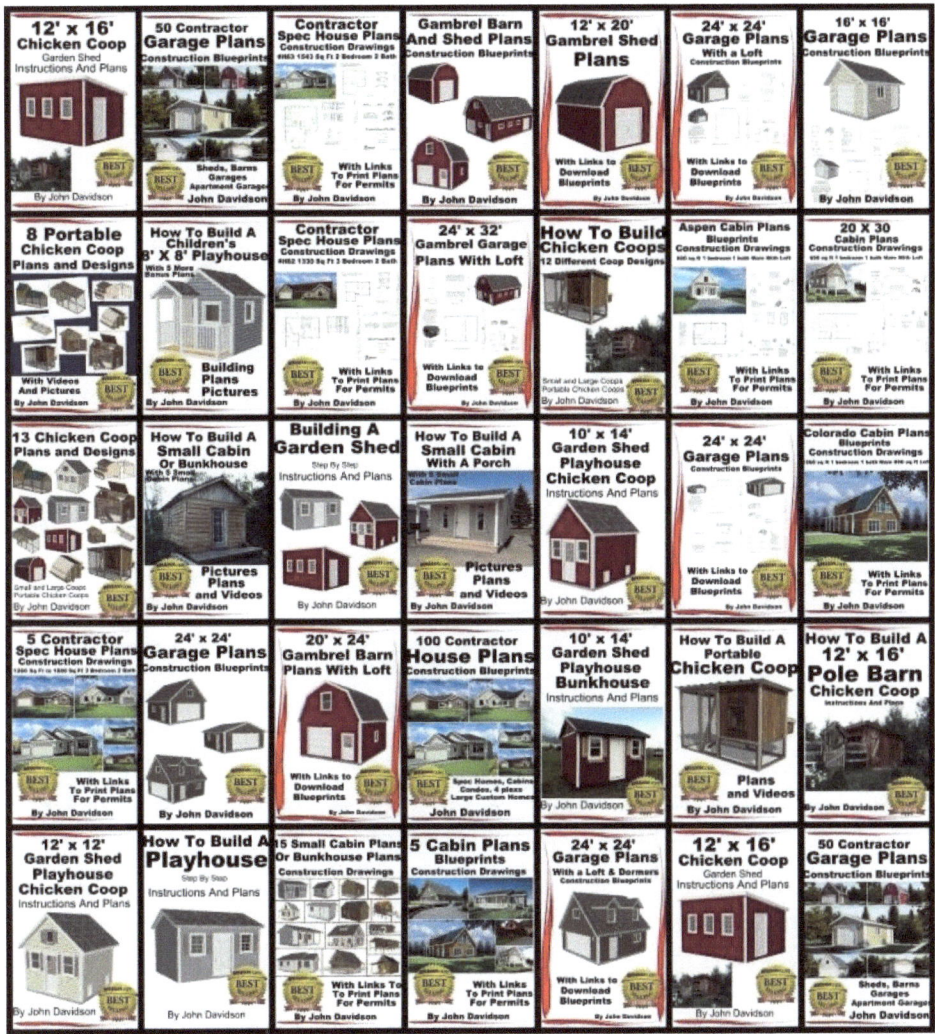

Entrepreneur Book Series

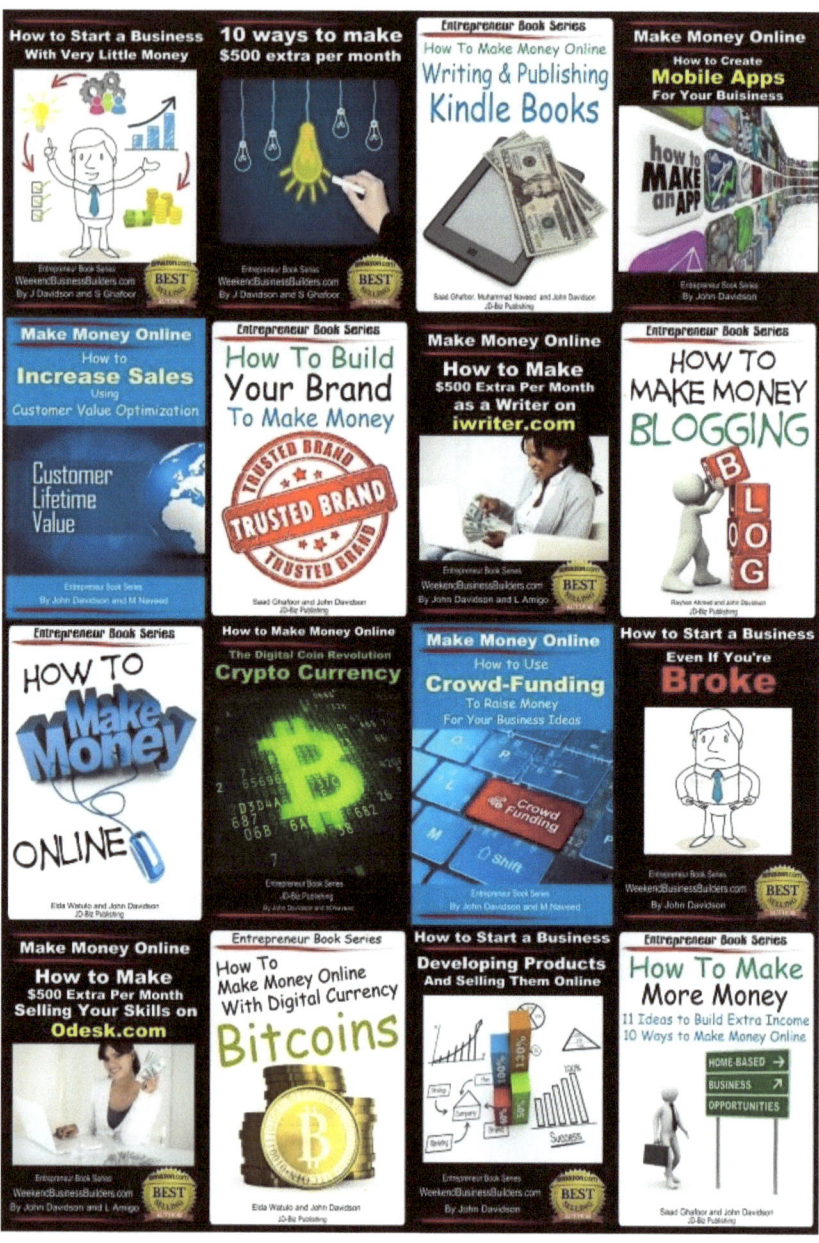

Our books are available at

1. Amazon.com

2. Barnes and Noble

3. Itunes

4. Kobo

5. Smashwords

6. Google Play Books

Download Free Books!

http://MendonCottageBooks.com

Publisher

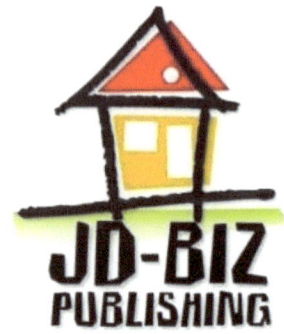

JD-Biz Corp

P O Box 374

Mendon, Utah 84325

http://www.jd-biz.com/

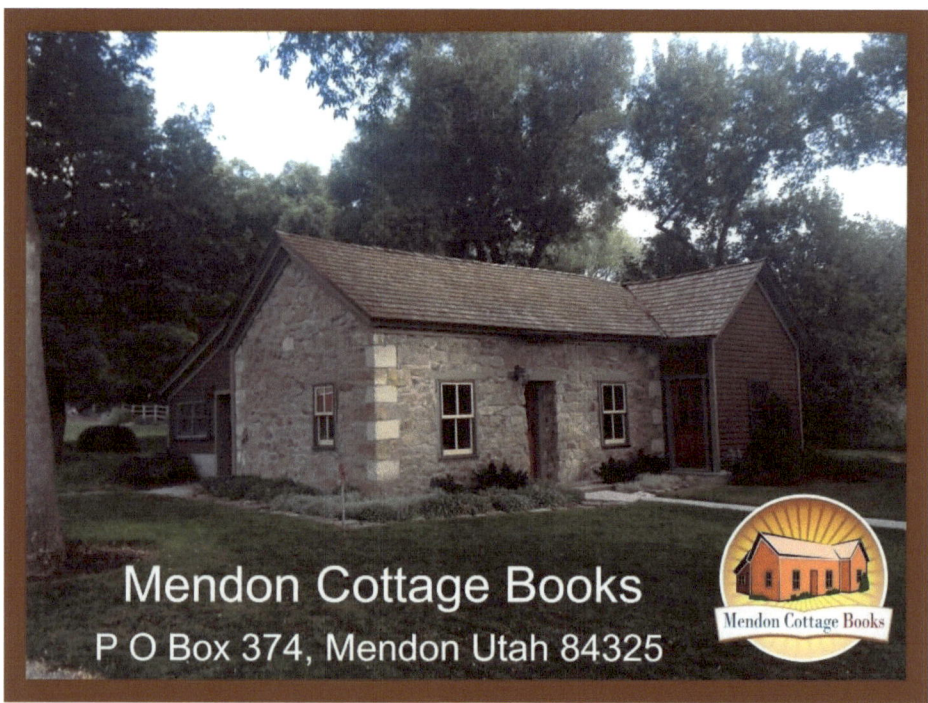

www.ingramcontent.com/pod-product-compliance
Lightning Source LLC
Chambersburg PA
CBHW050826290526
45792CB00001B/279